Table of Contents

An autoimmune disease is a condition in which your immune system attacks your body.

The immune system usually guards against bacteria and viruses. When it senses these foreign invaders, it sends out an army of fighter cells to attack them.

Usually, the immune system can tell the difference between foreign cells and your own cells.

In an autoimmune disease, the immune system mistakes part of your body, like your joints or skin, as foreign. It releases proteins called autoantibodies that attack healthy cells.

Some autoimmune diseases target only one organ. Type 1 diabetes damages the pancreas. Other diseases, like systemic lupus erythematosus (SLE), or lupus, can affect the whole body.

We've partnered with Cue Health, a healthcare company that makes lab-quality, portable diagnostic tests for at-home and professional use, to bring you this overview of autoimmune disease.

BREAKFAST

1. Sweet Potato & Turkey Hash

Prep Time: 5 Minutes

Cook Time: 30 Minutes

Servings: 4

Ingredients

- 1 tbsp coconut oil or avocado oil
- 1 lb ground turkey
- 1 medium sweet potato, diced
- 1.5 cups brussels sprouts, halved
- 1 pink lady apple, diced
- 2 cups kale, chopped
- 2 tsp rosemary
- 2 tsp sage
- 1 tsp sea salt

Instructions

1. Using a large cast iron skillet, or a pan, cook the ground turkey on medium heat until cooked through, lightly seasoning with some of the seasonings (reserve the majority for later). Set aside, reserving some of the fat in the pan.

2. Add in the coconut/avocado oil and saute the sweet potato for 5 minutes, before adding in the brussels sprouts. Saute for another 15 minutes until the veggies have softened and crisped to liking.

3. Add in the diced apple and kale and saute for another 4-5 minutes or until slightly softened.

4. Reincorporate the ground turkey, and add the remainder of the seasonings. Stir until fully combined, and season further to taste.

5. Serve warm and enjoy!

2. Plantain Waffles with Berry Compote

Prep Time: 10 Minutes

Cook Time: 25 Minutes

Servings: 4

Ingredients

Waffles:

- 3 plantains I use green ones but if you like sweeter waffles then use yellower ones
- 2 cups full fat coconut milk
- 1/3 cup melted coconut oil
- 2 eggs or 2 gelatin eggs use the gelatin eggs for AIP
- 1 tbsp vanilla extract omit for AIP
- 1/2 cup coconut flour
- 1 tsp baking soda
- 1/2 tsp sea salt

Berry Compote:

- 3 cups berries I used blueberries and raspberries this time but any berry should work

- 2 tbsp coconut oil

- 1/2 cup full fat coconut milk

- 1 tsp vanilla extract omit for AIP

- 1 tbsp arrowroot starch

Instructions

Waffle Instructions

1. Puree the plantains with 1 cup coconut milk in your food processor or high speed blender (NOTE: altogether this should yield 3 cups - depending on the size of your plantains you may need to add a little extra coconut milk).

2. Transfer the blended mixture to a mixing bowl and add the remaining coconut milk, coconut oil, eggs and vanilla extract and stir well until combined.

3. Add the dry ingredients and stir well until combined.

4. Turn on your waffle maker and let it heat up.

5. Transfer 1 cup of the batter to your waffle maker and cook for 5-6 minutes.

6. Continue until you use up all the batter. Then make the berry compote and serve!

Berry Compote Instructions

1. Place a medium pot on the stove on medium heat.
2. Add all the ingredients to the pot and let heat until bubbling.
3. Turn the heat down and simmer for 10-15 minutes to allow the berries to break apart.
4. Stir in the tapioca flour and cook for another 5 minutes.
5. Turn off the heat and let sit for a couple minutes to thicken.
6. Spoon the berry sauce over the waffles and enjoy!
7. To make a gelatin egg: combine 1 TBSP gelatin with 1 TBSP cold water and stir vigorously until the gelatin dissolves, then add 2 TBSP boiling water and beat well (it should make a frothy type substance).
8. Nutritional values are an estimate and will vary depending on the exact ingredients used.
9. If you don't want to make the berry compote you don't have to. You can serve these waffles with whatever you prefer.
10. Store these waffles in the fridge in an air tight container for up to 5 days.

3. Paleo Pumpkin Spice Pancake

Prep Time: 20 Minutes

Cook Time: 45 Minutes

Servings: 8

Ingredients

- 2 tablespoons gelatin
- 1/2 cup hot water
- 4 medjool dates, pits removed
- 1/2 cup pumpkin puree
- 2 tablespoons melted coconut oil
- 1 teaspoon apple cider vinegar
- 2/3 cup sweet potato flour
- 1 teaspoon baking soda
- 1/2 teaspoon salt
- 1 teaspoon cinnamon

Instructions

1. Preheat oven to 350°F and line a cookie sheet with parchment paper or a silicone mat.

2. Dissolve the gelatin in the hot water and mix well.

3. In a food processor or high speed blender, puree dates, pumpkin, coconut oil, apple cider vinegar, and the gelatin and water mixture until smooth.

4. Add sweet potato flour, baking soda, salt and cinnamon. Puree again until all ingredients are well combined (the batter will be thick – more like a cake than a traditional pancake).

5. Make six roughly equal size pancakes on the cookie sheet – spreading them out so that each one is about 1/4 inch thick.

6. Bake for 25-30 minutes, or until they hold together when you gently slide a spatula under them and try to move them.

7. Serve with desired topping (maple syrup, honey, or coconut cream) or eat plain.

4. Sunrise Beef Hash

Prep Time: 25 Minutes

Cook Time: 50 Minutes

Servings: 4

Ingredients

- 1 tablespoon coconut oil or other fat
- 1 small onion, chopped
- 2 cloves garlic
- 1/2 teaspoon cinnamon
- 1 teaspoon ginger
- 1 teaspoon turmeric
- 1/2 teaspoon salt
- 1 pound ground beef (preferably grass fed)
- 1–2 medium sweet potatoes, peeled and cut into small cubes
- 1 bunch (about 10 ounces) kale, chopped into bite sized pieces
- 1 tablespoon lemon juice

Instructions

1. In a cast iron skillet, heat coconut oil over medium heat. Add onions and cook until softened and becoming translucent (about 5 minutes).
2. Stir in garlic, cinnamon, ginger, turmeric, and salt. Cook until fragrant (about 1 minute) and then immediately add ground beef. Break up beef as it cooks with a wooden spoon and stir as needed.
3. When beef is just barely cooked through add sweet potatoes and cook, continuing to stir frequently, until potatoes are softened (about 5-7 more minutes).
4. Stir in kale and allow to cook until wilted and softened (about 3 minutes). Check sweet potatoes for doneness – if they are not as soft as you desire, cook longer.
5. Stir in lemon juice. Taste and add more salt if desired.

5. Green Breakfast Soup

Prep Time: 30 Minutes

Cook Time: 1hrs 50 Minutes

Servings: 8-10

Ingredients

- 1 large, whole pastured chicken (5–6 pounds)
- 1 bay leaf
- 1 tablespoon apple cider vinegar
- 1 tablespoon sea salt, plus additional to taste
- 2 tablespoons solid cooking fat
- 1 onion, chopped
- 4 cloves garlic, minced
- 1/3 cup peeled and minced fresh ginger (3- to 4- inch piece)
- 2 large sweet potatoes, chopped into 1 1/2 inch chunks (about 6 cups)
- 2 large zucchini, chopped into 1 1/2 inch chunks (about 2 cups)
- 1 bunch Swiss chard, stems and leaves divided and chopped

- 2 cups button mushrooms, thinly sliced
- 1 bunch green onions (ends removed), thinly sliced, for serving
- 1 lemon, cut into wedges, for serving

Instructions

1. Begin by cleaning the chicken (rinse it under cold water and remove loose bits of fat and other tissue). Place it in a large stock pot. If it doesn't fit, you will have to cut it into halves or quarters (kitchen shears help here — start by cutting up one side of the backbone).
2. Add the bay leaf, vinegar, and 1 tablespoon sea salt. Fill the pot with cold water until the chicken is just covered. Bring to a boil, and then cover tightly and lower the heat to a bare simmer. Cook until the meat is tender and falling off the bone, 60 to 90 minutes – the lower the simmer, the more tender the chicken will come out. Skim the surface of the broth to remove any scum that may appear during cooking.
3. Remove the chicken from the pot and set aside to cool. Pour the broth through a fine-mesh strainer,

being careful to save the broth in another pot! Discard the bay leaf.

4. Place the empty pot back on the stove, add the solid cooking fat, and turn the heat to medium. When the fat has melted and the pan is hot, add the onions and cook, stirring, for 7 minutes, or until translucent. Add the garlic and ginger and cook, stirring, for another few minutes, until fragrant.

5. While the onions are cooking, remove the meat from the chicken carcass, shred it with two forks (CAUTION: hot!), and set it aside in the bowl. Keep the bones to add to your next batch of bone broth.

6. Add the sweet potatoes and broth back to the pot, bring to a boil, and then cover and turn down to a simmer. Cook for 10 minutes.

7. Add the zucchini, chard stems, and mushrooms, and cook for another 5 minutes, or until the vegetables are tender. Turn off the heat and stir in the chard leaves.

8. Carefully transfer half of the soup to a blender, blend for 30 seconds, and transfer back to the pot. Alternatively, you could use an immersion blender to blend about half of the vegetables (CAUTION: Make sure you have a blender that can handle hot liquid,

and make sure to use a towel above the lid to protect your hands from getting burned.)

9. Return the blended liquid to the soup pot, with the chicken. Add salt to taste.

10. Serve each bowl garnished with green onions and a squeeze of fresh lemon juice.

6. Beef and Mushroom Parsnip Risotto

Prep Time: 25 Minutes

Cook Time: 50 Minutes

Servings: 5

Ingredients

- 1 Tbsp evoo
- 1 carrot, diced
- 1/2 medium white onion, diced
- 1 lb groud beef
- 8 oz cremini mushrooms, sliced
- 2 cups (1 box) Kettle & Fire Beef Broth, divided
- 1 Tbsp apple cider vinegar or 1/4 cup wine (red or white)
- 1 1/2 tsp salt, plus more to taste
- 2 lbs parsnips (6-7 cups riced)
- 1 Tbsp finely chopped fresh tarragon (1 tsp dried tarragon)
- 1/2 cup full fat coconut milk

Instructions

1. To rice parsnips: Peel parsnips and chop into big chunks. Place in a food processor and pulse until pieces are fairly uniform in size and about the size of a large grain of rice. Two pounds of parsnips (about 5-6 medium parsnips) should yield 6-7 cups once riced.

2. Heat a large skillet over medium-high heat. Add olive oil, onion and carrot. Saute until veggies are tender, about 5 minutes.

3. Add ground beef to skillet and cook, stirring to break up the beef, until browned, about 3-5 minutes.

4. Add mushrooms, 1 cup of broth, wine (or vinegar) and salt. Increase heat to high and cook until the liquid is mostly evaporated, 5-8 minutes.

5. Add parsnips and remaining 1 cup of broth to pan and stir just to mix. Reduce heat to medium-low, and cover. Cook 8-10 minutes until parsnips are tender and mushy, stirring once or twice during that cooking time. If veggies start to stick because the pan is running dry, add another few tablespoons of broth or water to the pan. If you're largest skillet isn't big enough for all of these ingredients, you can remove the beef mixture before adding the parsnips and then mix the beef mixture back in right before serving.

6. Add coconut milk and tarragon and stir to incorporate. Turn off the heat and let sit on the stovetop covered for 2-3 minutes more. Taste and add additional salt, if needed.

7. Garnish with chopped parsley if desired. Serve!

7. Paleo One-Pan Beef and Broccoli

Prep Time: 15 Minutes

Cook Time: 20 Minutes

Servings: 4

Ingredients

- 1 head of broccoli (1 lb or 450 g), broken into small florets
- 2 Tablespoons (30 ml) avocado oil, to cook with
- 1 cloves of garlic, peeled and minced
- 1 teaspoon (2 g) fresh ginger, peeled and minced
- 1lb (450 g) flank steak, thinly sliced
- 3 Tablespoons (45 ml) coconut aminos
- 1 Tablespoon (15 g) coconut sugar (optional)
- 6 Tablespoons (90 ml) water, divided (plus additional to steam broccoli)
- 1 Tablespoon (15 ml) lime juice
- 1 teaspoon (2 g) xanthan gum
- 1 teaspoon (5 g) sesame seeds, for garnish
- Salt and pepper, to taste

Instructions

1. Heat a large skillet on the stove over medium-high heat. Add the broccoli and 1-inch (2 ½ cm) of water to the skillet. Cover and steam the broccoli for about 2 minutes. Remove the lid and drain any excess liquid.

2. Add the avocado oil, garlic and fresh ginger to the skillet and saute until fragrant, about 2 minutes.

3. Add the sliced steak, coconut aminos and optional coconut sugar to the skillet and saute for 3 to 5 minutes.

4. Add 4 Tablespoons (60 ml) of water and lime juice to the skillet to deglaze the pan, using a wooden spoon to scrape the browned bits from the bottom of the skillet, and continue to saute for about 2 minutes.

5. Meanwhile, in a small bowl, whisk to combine the xanthan gum and the remaining 2 Tablespoons (30 ml) of water until smooth with no lumps remaining.

6. While constantly stirring, pour the xanthan mixture into the skillet and continue to stir until the sauce is thick to your liking. Season with salt and pepper, to taste.

7. Garnish the beef and broccoli with the sesame seeds and serve immediately.

8. Paleo Spaghetti with Tomato Sauce

Prep Time: 15 Minutes

Cook Time: 20 Minutes

Servings: 4

Ingredients

- ½ small onion, chopped
- 1 can (14 oz) diced tomatoes
- 2 Tablespoons Italian seasoning
- 1 bell pepper, chopped
- 1 zucchini, chopped
- 4 cloves of garlic, minced
- ¼ cup basil, chopped (for garnish)
- Olive oil to cook in
- Salt and pepper to taste
- 2 teaspoons honey (optional – omit for keto)

For the pasta

- 1 large cucumber, peeled

Instructions

1. In a saucepan, saute the chopped onion in olive oil until translucent. Add in the diced tomatoes, Italian seasoning, bell pepper, and zucchini. Cook until the bell pepper and zucchini have softened.

2. Meanwhile, peel a large cucumber and then use the peeler to create strands out of the cucumber. Divide into 2 large bowls.

3. Add the minced garlic, basil, and salt and pepper to the tomato sauce and pour the sauce on top of the cucumber pasta.

9. Apple & Cranberry Paleo Oatmeal

Prep Time: 20 Minutes

Cook Time: 45 Minutes

Servings: 4

Ingredients

- 1 medium-large acorn squash
- 2 cups / 480 ml coconut milk
- 3/4 cup / 60 g unsweetened shredded coconut
- 1 cup / 215 g peeled & grated apple (about 2)
- 1 cup / 80 g fresh or frozen cranberries, roughly chopped
- 1/2 tsp ground cinnamon
- 1/4 tsp fine sea salt
- Optional, to serve: pure maple syrup or raw honey

Instructions

Roast:

1. Preheat the oven to 400 F / 205 C. Carefully cut the acorn squash in half, then scoop out the seeds. Cover the bottom of a 7 x 11 baking dish with water, then place the acorn squash halves, cut side down, into the dish. Roast until the squash is tender, about 45 minutes. Remove from the oven and allow to cool.

Simmer:

2. When the cooked squash is cool enough to handle, scoop out 2 cups / 400 g of the flesh and add it to a medium sized saucepan. Add all other ingredients to the pan over medium heat and bring almost to an even simmer, stirring to combine the ingredients evenly. Reduce the heat a little to maintain an gentle simmer and cook, stirring occasionally, until the apple and cranberries have softened and the oatmeal has thickened, about 20 minutes. Serve drizzled with a little maple syrup or raw honey, if you like. I like to finish mine off with some extra chopped apples as a nice crunchy topping, too!

10. Paleo Egg Roll in a Bowl

Prep Time: 15 Minutes

Cook Time: 20 Minutes

Servings: 4

Ingredients

- 2 Tablespoons (30 ml) avocado oil
- 1/2 medium onion (2 oz or 55 g), chopped
- 2 cloves of garlic (6 g), peeled and minced
- 1 lb (450 g) ground pork
- 1 teaspoon (5 g) salt
- 1/2 teaspoon (1 g) pepper
- 1/2 teaspoon (1 g) onion powder
- 1/2 teaspoon (1 g) ginger powder
- 1 package (14 oz or 400 g) coleslaw mix
- 1/2 cup (120 ml) gluten-free tamari sauce or coconut aminos
- 1 Tablespoon (15 ml) honey (if using gluten-free tamari sauce)
- Red pepper flakes, for garnish (optional)

Instructions

3. Add the avocado oil to a large skillet over medium-high heat. Add the onion and garlic to the skillet and saute until the onion is translucent.

4. Add the ground pork, salt, pepper, onion powder and ginger powder to the skillet and saute until the ground pork is browned.

5. Add the coleslaw mix, tamari sauce or coconut aminos and honey (if using tamari sauce) and continue to cook until the ground pork is cooked through and the vegetables cooked to your liking.

6. If desired, garnish with the egg roll in a bowl with red pepper flakes and serve immediately.

11. Keto Sweet and Sour Chicken

Prep Time: 10 Minutes

Cook Time: 15 Minutes

Servings:

Ingredients

Sweet and Sour Sauce

- 7 oz tomato paste
- 1 1/2 cups chicken bone broth
- 1/3 cup swerve
- 1/4 cup coconut vinegar
- 1 tablespoon lime juice
- 3/4 tablespoon fish sauce
- 1/2 teaspoon sea salt
- 1/2 teaspoon garlic powder
- 1/8 teaspoon ginger, fresh grated
- 1/4 teaspoon guar gum, (optional)

Chicken

- 1 cup coconut oil, for frying

- 2 large eggs

- 1 1/2 cups powdered parmesan cheese

- 1/4 teaspoon black pepper

- 1 lb boneless, skinless chicken thighs, cut into bite-sized pieces

- scallions, slices, for garnish

Instructions

1. Keto Sweet and Sour Sauce - Use only 1/4 Cup for the recipe

2. Place the tomato paste, broth, sweetener, vinegar, lime juice, fish sauce, salt, garlic powder and ginger in a medium-zied saucepan over medium heat. Stir well to combine. Bring the mixture to a boil, stirring often. Boil for 3 minutes, stirring occasionally, until thickened to your liking. Remove from the heat and let cool. Sift in the guar gum, if using, and whisk until well combined. Pour the sauce into a jar and refrigerate until ready to use.

Chicken

1. Heat the oil in a 4-inch-deep (or deeper) cast-iron skillet over medium heat at 350 degrees. The oil should be 1 inch deep, add more if needed.

2. Bread the chicken: Crack the eggs into a shallow baking dish and beat lightly with a fork. In another shallow baking dish, combine the powdered Parmesan and pepper. Dip a chicken nugget into the eggs, then the cheese mixture. Coat well.

3. When the oil is hot, fry the nuggets in batches for about 5 minutes, until golden brown and cooked through.

4. Baste the fried chicken nuggets with the sauce. Serve over cauliflower rice and garnish with scallions, if desired

12. Keto Chicken Fried Rice

Prep Time: 10 Minutes

Cook Time: 20 Minutes

Servings: 4

Ingredients

- 3 tbsp unsalted butter divided
- 2 large eggs lightly beaten
- Sea salt and black pepper to taste
- 1 lb boneless, skinless chicken breast, cut into 1/2" pieces
- 2 cups frozen riced cauliflower
- 1/4 cup frozen peas and carrots mixture
- 1 large green onion sliced
- 1 tsp fresh ginger finely minced
- 1/2 tsp garlic powder
- 1/2 tsp crushed red pepper flakes or to taste
- 1-2 tsp Swerve or erythritol optional
- 3 tbsp tamari or coconut aminos
- 2 tbsp toasted sesame oil

Instructions

1. Heat 1 tbsp butter in a wok or large high-sided skillet over medium-high heat. Add eggs and season with salt and pepper to taste. Cook, stirring constantly, for 1-2 minutes or until eggs are cooked through. Transfer eggs to a plate and set aside.

2. Add 1 tbsp butter, diced chicken breasts, and half of the ginger, half of the garlic powder, and half of the red pepper flakes to the hot wok or skillet. Season with salt and pepper to taste. Cook for 4-6 minutes, stirring frequently until the chicken is cooked through. Transfer chicken to a plate and set aside.

3. Again add 1 tbsp butter to the hot wok or skillet, plus the frozen cauliflower, peas and carrots, green onions, Swerve or erythritol (optional), and remaining ginger, garlic powder, and red pepper flakes. Season with salt and pepper to taste. Cook, stirring frequently until the frozen veggies are heated through and tender, approximately 3-5 minutes.

4. Finally, to the cooked vegetable mixture, add tamari (or coconut aminos), sesame oil, cooked eggs, and cooked chicken. Cook for 1-2 minutes, stirring constantly, or until all ingredients are thoroughly combined and heated through. Remove your keto

chicken fried rice from heat and top with additional green onion, if desired, and serve immediately.

5. If you don't like a lot of heat, reduce or eliminate the crushed red pepper flakes. If you love heat, maintain or increase the called-for amount.

6. Tamari is lower in carbs than coconut aminos; using coconut aminos will add an extra 1.5g net carbs per serving of this dish if you use a full 3 tbsp coconut aminos (Coconut Secret brand). Nutrition facts have been calculated based on the usage of tamari.

13. Chicken Pad Thai

Prep Time: 10 Minutes

Cook Time: 20 Minutes

Servings: 4

Ingredients

Sauce:

- 3 tablespoon fish sauce
- 1 tablespoon rice vinegar
- 1 tablespoon sambal oelek (chili paste, use 1 teaspoon if you prefer less heat)
- 1 tablespoon peanut butter
- 1 tablespoon coconut aminos
- 2 tablespoon lime juice
- 5 drops stevia

Keto Pad Thai:

- 1 16 oz package shirataki noodles
- 1 lb chicken breast, butterflied and cut into bit sized pieces
- 2 eggs, beaten

- ½ tablespoon ginger, minced
- 2 cloves garlic, minced
- 3 large scallions, thinly sliced, keep whites and greens separate
- 1 tablespoon sambal oelek
- 1 ½ cups bean sprouts

Toppings:

- ¼ cup peanuts, chopped
- ⅓ cup cilantro leaves, chopped

Instructions

1. Wash and dry fresh produce. Thinly slice scallions, keeping whites and greens separated. Peel and mince ginger and garlic. Roughly chop cilantro leaves.
2. Butterfly the chicken breast then cut into small bite sized pieces.
3. In a small bowl, whisk together all sauce ingredients until well combined and smooth.
4. Heat a drizzle of oil (I used sesame oil) in a wok or large pan over medium high heat. Add ginger and garlic and stir fry until fragrant (about 30 seconds),

stirring frequently. Add scallion whites and 1 tablespoon sambal oelek to wok with ginger and garlic and continue stir frying until scallions have softened about 2-3 minutes.

5. Once scallion whites have softened, add chicken to wok with the ginger, garlic, scallions, and sambal oelek. Stir fry chicken for 5 minutes or until lightly browned and cooked through.

6. While chicken cooks, beat 2 eggs until well combined. Drain and rinse shirataki noodles thoroughly under hot water for about 2 minutes.

7. Once chicken has finished, remove the chicken stir fry the wok or pan and set aside. Add shiratki noodles to the wok and stir fry noodles until firm, about 5-7 minutes.

8. Once noodles have cooked, add the beaten eggs to the wok with the noodles and stir fry for 2-3 minutes until the eggs have cooked. Stir frequently to break up/scramble the eggs.

9. Once eggs have cooked, add the chicken stir fry, pad thai sauce, and bean sprouts to the wok. Continue stir frying for about 2 minutes until all ingredients are well combined.

10. Top with scallion greens, crushed peanuts, and cilantro to serve. Enjoy!

14. Asian Beef Bowl

Prep Time: 10 Minutes

Cook Time: 20 Minutes

Servings: 4

Ingredients

- 1 pound ground beef or pork (full fat)
- 1 bunch greens of green onions , chopped (reserve some for garnish)
- ¼ cup sesame oil , toasted, or preferred traditional fat (lard, avocado oil, coconut oil, bacon fat for AIP)
- ¼ cup fresh ginger , minced or grated
- 2 Tablespoons soy sauce , real fermented OR for Paleo, GAPS, Whole30, AIP - ¼ cup coconut amino acids
- 5 cloves garlic minced or crushed
- 1/16 teaspoon powdered stevia , (omit for Whole30) or to taste, brands vary considerably; or use 15-20 drops of liquid stevia, to taste; or sub 2 Tablespoons honey for AIP and GAPS

- sesame seeds and prepared cauliflower rice, for serving (omit for AIP)

Instructions

1. In large cast iron skillet or wok, cook green onions in sesame oil over medium-high heat until they begin to soften and brown, about 4 to 5 minutes.
2. Add beef and, with metal/wooden spatula, break up into smaller pieces continually, cooking until the outside is no longer pink, about 8 minutes.
3. Add soy sauce or coconut amino acids, ginger, garlic and stevia. Simmer 2 to 3 minutes, stirring in the new ingredients.
4. Serve on top of hot, cooked cauli rice, garnished with sesame seeds and green onions' greens or fresh cilantro/chives etc.

15. Southern-Style Cornmeal Catfish with Tomato Gravy

Prep Time: 25 Minutes

Cook Time: 55 Minutes

Servings: 4

Ingredients

- 2 Tbsp rendered bacon fat
- 2 Tbsp plus ½ cup ground cornmeal
- 1 can (14.5oz) whole peeled tomatoes, lightly crushed, juices discarded
- Salt and black pepper to taste
- 1 Tbsp canola oil
- ⅛ tsp cayenne pepper
- 4 catfish fillets (about 6 oz each)

Instructions

1. Heat the bacon fat in a medium saucepan over low heat.

2. Add the 2 tablespoons of cornmeal and continue cooking, stirring constantly, for about 5 minutes, until the cornmeal is light brown.

3. Add the drained tomatoes and simmer for another 10 minutes. Season with salt and black pepper.

4. While the sauce simmers, prepare the catfish: Heat the oil in a large cast-iron skillet or non-stick pan over medium heat.

5. Spread the ½ cup of cornmeal out in a shallow dish and season with the cayenne, plus a few good pinches of salt and black pepper.

6. Dust the catfish on both sides with the cornmeal and place in the hot pan.

7. Cook, turning once, for 6 to 8 minutes, until the surface is golden brown and crusty and the fish flakes with gentle pressure from your finger.

8. Serve each fillet with a big scoop of tomato gravy.

16. Warm Goat Cheese Salad

Prep Time: 25 Minutes

Cook Time: 55 Minutes

Servings: 4

Ingredients

- 1 log (4 oz) fresh goat cheese
- 1 cup bread crumbs
- 1 tsp dried thyme or Italian seasoning
- Salt and black pepper to taste
- 1 egg, lightly beaten
- 1/4 cup walnuts
- 16 cups mixed greens or arugula (6-oz bag)
- Balsamic vinaigrette
- 1 pear, peeled, cored, and sliced

Instructions

1. Slice the goat cheese into four 1/2" disks (a piece of unflavored dental floss makes this job easy).

2. If the cheese crumbles, use your hands to form it back into disks.

3. Pour the bread crumbs onto a plate and toss with the thyme and a pinch each of salt and pepper.

4. Dip the goat cheese into the egg, then into the crumb mixture and turn to coat evenly.

5. Place the disks on a plate and into the freezer for 15 minutes to firm up.

6. Preheat the oven to 450°F.

7. Place the goat cheese on a baking sheet coated with non-stick cooking spray and bake for 10 minutes, until the cheese is soft and the crumbs are toasted.

8. Remove. While the oven is still hot, toast the walnuts for 5 minutes.

9. Toss the lettuce with the vinaigrette and pear. Divide among 4 cold plates. Top with the walnuts and goat cheese.

Fresh Goat Cheese

1. Break free from the reliance on cheddar and mozzarella and discover some of the truly fantastic cheeses that too many serious eaters overlook. Fresh goat cheese has a tangy creaminess that makes it one of the most versatile in the dairy case, great for crumbling onto salads, spreading on sandwiches, or

folding into warm pasta dishes. Our favorite goat cheeses are made by Cypress Grove Chevre and are available in supermarkets nationwide. An ounce has just 70 calories and 6 grams of fat, making it one of the healthiest cheeses you'll find.

17. Scallops with Chimichurri

Prep Time: 20 Minutes

Cook Time: 60 Minutes

Servings: 3

Ingredients

- ½ cup water with salt
- 2 Tbsp red wine vinegar
- cup fresh parsley, chopped
- cloves garlic, minced
- Pinch red pepper flakes
- Tbsp olive oil
- 1 lb large sea scallops
- Black pepper to taste

Instructions

1. Combine the water and ½ teaspoon salt in a bowl and microwave for 30 seconds. Stir so the salt thoroughly dissolves, then mix in the vinegar, parsley, garlic, and pepper flakes.

2. Slowly drizzle in 2 tablespoons of the olive oil, whisking to incorporate. You can use the chimichurri now, but it's best to let the flavors marry for 20 minutes or more; it will keep covered in the fridge for 3 days.

3. Heat the remaining 1 tablespoon oil in a large skillet over medium-high heat. Thoroughly dry the scallops with paper towels, then season on both sides with salt and pepper.

4. When the oil is hot, add the scallops and cook for 2 to 3 minutes on the first side, without disturbing them, until a deep brown crust has developed. Flip and cook for 1 to 2 minutes longer, until firm but yielding to the touch. Serve drizzled with the chimichurri.

18. Scallops with White Beans and Spinach

Prep Time: 10 Minutes

Cook Time: 25 Minutes

Servings: 3

Ingredients

- 2 strips bacon, chopped into small pieces (Feel free to kill the bacon, but for about 18 calories per serving, it adds a ton of flavor to the overall dish.)
- ½ red onion, minced
- clove garlic, minced
- 1 can (14 oz) white beans, rinsed and drained (There are a lot of different types of white beans sold in cans. All will work, but cannellini beans are best.)
- 4 cups baby spinach
- 1 lb large sea scallops
- Salt and black pepper to taste
- 1 Tbsp butter
- Juice of 1 lemon

Instructions

1. Heat a medium saucepan over low heat.
2. Cook the bacon until it has begun to crisp.
3. Add the onion and garlic; saute until the onion is soft and translucent, 2 to 3 minutes.
4. Add the beans and spinach and simmer until the beans are hot and the spinach is wilted. Keep warm.
5. Heat a large cast-iron skillet or saute pan over medium-high heat.
6. Blot the scallops dry with a paper towel and season with salt and pepper on both sides.
7. Add the butter and the scallops to the pan and sear the scallops for 2 to 3 minutes per side, until deeply caramelized.
8. Before serving, add the lemon juice to the beans.
9. Season with salt and pepper.
10. Divide the beans among 4 warm bowls or plates and top with scallops.

19. innamon-Roasted Sweet Potato Salad with Wild Rice

Prep Time: 20 Minutes

Cook Time: 60 Minutes

Servings: 4

Ingredients

- 12 oz sweet potato, scrubbed and cut into 1/2-inch pieces
- 1medium red or yellow onion, sliced into wedges
- 4 Tbsp olive oil
- 1 tsp salt
- 1/2 tsp black pepper
- 1/4 tsp ground cinnamon
- 2 Tbsp rice wine vinegar
- 1 Tbsp curry powder
- 2tsp honey
- 1/2 tsp salt
- 1/4 tsp black pepper
- 2cups cooked wild rice

- 4oz cooked chicken, shredded
- 1/4 cup golden or regular raisins
- 2 medium carrots, shaved
- 1/4 cup snipped fresh cilantro

Instructions

1. Preheat oven to 400°F. Line a baking sheet with foil, and coat with cooking spray.
2. In a medium bowl, combine sweet potato, onion, 1 Tbsp oil, 1/2 tsp salt, 1/4 tsp pepper, and cinnamon; toss to coat. Transfer potato mixture to prepared baking sheet. Roast about 20 minutes or until tender.
3. Meanwhile, in a small bowl, combine remaining 3 Tbsp oil, vinegar, curry powder, honey, the remaining 1/2 tsp salt, and the remaining 1/4 tsp pepper. Whisk until smooth.
4. Divide rice among four pint jars. Top with roasted potatoes, chicken, raisins, and carrots. Drizzle with dressing and top with cilantro. Cover and chill up to 3 days.
5. Wild rice has nearly double the fiber and protein and fewer calories than brown rice.

20. Cooker Cuban Tomato and Black Bean Soup

Prep Time: 25 Minutes

Cook Time: 55 Minutes

Servings: 6

Ingredients

- 2 15-ounce cans reduced-sodium black beans, rinsed and drained
- 1 32-ounce carton unsalted chicken broth
- 1 14.5-ounce can no-salt-added diced tomatoes
- 1 smoked ham hock
- 1 cup chopped onions
- 1 medium red sweet pepper, 1 medium fresh jalapeño pepper, seeded (if desired) and finely chopped
- 1/4 cup orange juice
- 2 cloves
- 1 Tbsp cider vinegar
- 1 tsp ground cumin
- 1 tsp dried oregano, crushed

- 1/4 tsp salt
- 1/4 tsp black pepper
- Plain fat-free Greek yogurt
- Sliced green onions
- Lime wedge

Instructions

1. In a small mixing bowl, mash one can of beans until nearly smooth. In a 4- to 6-quart slow cooker, combine the mashed beans, whole beans, and the next 13 ingredients (through black pepper). Cover and cook on low 6 to 8 hours or on high 3 to 4 hours.
2. Remove ham hock. If desired, cut meat from bone and return meat to soup; discard bone.
3. Top with yogurt and sprinkle with green onions. Serve with lime wedges for squeezing.

21. Spinach Salad Topped with Goat Cheese, Apples, and Warm Bacon Dressing

Prep Time: 25 Minutes

Cook Time: 55 Minutes

Servings: 6

Ingredients

- 6 strips bacon, chopped
- 1 small red onion, sliced
- 1 green apple, peeled and sliced
- 1/4 cup pecans
- 2 Tbsp red wine vinegar
- 1 Tbsp Dijon mustard
- 1 Tbsp olive oil
- Salt and black pepper to taste
- 1 bunch spinach, washed, dried, and stemmed
- 1/4 cup fresh goat cheese

Instructions

1. Heat a large cast-iron skillet or nonstick pan over medium heat.
2. Add the bacon and cook for about 5 minutes, until browned and just crisp.
3. Remove to a paper towel-lined plate and reserve.
4. Add the onion to the same pan and cook for 2 to 3 minutes, until just soft.
5. Add the apple and pecans and continue sautéing for 2 minutes, until the pecans are lightly toasted and the apple softened.
6. Add the vinegar, mustard, and olive oil, along with a few pinches of salt and plenty of black pepper.
7. Use a wooden spoon to stir the mixture vigorously to help it emulsify into a unified dressing.
8. Divide the spinach and goat cheese among 4 bowls and pour the warm dressing directly over the greens. Garnish with the reserved bacon.

22.Restaurant-WorthyJalapeño Cheeseburger

Prep Time: 15 Minutes

Cook Time: 35 Minutes

Servings: 2

Ingredients

- 2 Tbsp ketchup
- 2 Tbsp relish
- 1 Tbsp olive oil mayonnaise
- Salt and black pepper
- 1 lb ground sirloin
- 1 cup shredded Pepper Jack cheese
- 1 cup caramelized onions
- ¼ cup pickled jalapeños
- 4 potato buns, split

Instructions

1. Combine the ketchup, relish, and mayo in a mixing bowl. Season with a pinch of salt and pepper and set aside.
2. Preheat a grill, grill pan, or cast-iron skillet.
3. Combine the ground sirloin with ½ teaspoon salt and ½ teaspoon pepper and mix gently.
4. Without overworking the meat, form into four patties until the beef just comes together.
5. When the grill or skillet is hot (if using a skillet, add a touch of oil), add the patties.
6. Cook on the first side for 5 to 6 minutes, until a nice crust develops.
7. Flip and immediately top with the cheese. Cook for another 2 to 3 minutes, until the cheese is melted and the burgers are firm but still yielding to the touch.
8. Remove the burgers.
9. While the grill or pan is hot, toast the buns.
10. Slather the bottom buns with the reserved spread, then top each with a burger, caramelized onions, and pickled jalapeños.
11. Crown with the bun tops and serve.
12. If you like burgers as much as we do, it's important to find the right bun for the base of your next

masterpiece. We love potato buns, not just because their squishy, compact size holds a 4-ounce patty perfectly, but because they tend to deliver a good dose of fiber for a light caloric toll.

13. Take our favorite burger vessel, For 130 calories you get 2 grams of fiber and 7 grams of protein. Compare that with whole-wheat buns, many of which pack 150 or more calories, and you'll see why we love the humble spud rolls so much.

23. Cheeseburger Casserole

Prep Time: 20 Minutes

Cook Time: 45 Minutes

Servings: 8

Ingredients

- 1Tbsp olive oil
- 3lb ground beef
- 1medium white onion, chopped
- 1tsp garlic powder
- 1tsp onion powder
- 1tsp kosher salt
- Freshly ground black pepper
- 1/4 cup tomato paste
- 1/4 cup Rao's Marinara Sauce
- 1 1/2 cups heavy cream
- 1 1/4 cup shredded Colby jack cheese
- 1/4 cup chopped chives

Instructions

1. Preheat oven to 375°F.

2. In a very large, shallow pan, heat the oil and add the ground beef. Use a metal pancake turner to press the beef down into a single layer that covers the entire surface of the pan. Cook for 5 to 7 minutes until browned, then use the pancake turner to flip the beef over and cook for another few minutes. Use a large spoon to spoon out excess liquid, until only a small amount remains.

3. Add onion, garlic powder, onion powder, salt, pepper, and tomato paste to the beef. Stir and cook for 1 minute. Add marinara sauce and heavy cream and remove from heat.

4. Stir in 1 cup of shredded cheese and spoon the beef mix into a large casserole dish.

5. Top with remaining cheese and bake about 10 minutes until the cheese is bubbling and melty. Top with chives and serve immediately

24. Low-Calorie Chicago Hot Dog

Prep Time: 15 Minutes

Cook Time: 60 Minutes

Servings: 3

Ingredients

- 4reduced-fat all-beef dogs
- 4poppy seed hot dog buns
- Yellow mustard relish
- 1small yellow onion, minced
- 1large beefsteak tomato, cut into wedges
- 4pickle spears
- 8sport peppers (These little light green chiles have an awesome spicy pop but are tough to come by. Pepperoncini, if need be, can fill in.)
- Celery salt

Instructions

1. Bring a medium pot of water to boil.

2. Turn the heat to low, add the hot dogs, and cook for 5 minutes, until heated all the way through.

3. Alternatively, you can grill the dogs until lightly charred all over (which, while untraditional, is probably more delicious).

4. Dump out all but a few inches of the water and place a steamer basket in the pot. Steam the buns until warm and very soft.

5. Place a dog in each bun, then arrange the toppings in the following order: mustard, relish, onion, a few tomato wedges, pickle spear, two sport peppers, and a pinch of celery salt.

6. Chicagoans are particular about their ingredients: The buns must be poppy seed, the relish must be neon green (often called piccalilli), and the peppers must be sport peppers. Finding all of that in your local market is next to impossible. If you want a 100 percent authentic Chicago dog, you can pick up all the authentic fixings at Vienna Beef, or you can do what we do and wing it.

25. Hot Ham and Cheese Sandwich with Chipotle Mayo

Prep Time: 30 Minutes

Cook Time: 55 Minutes

Servings: 3

Ingredients

For the mayo:

- 1/2 cup light mayonnaise
- 2 chipotle chiles in adobo sauce
- 1 Tbsp adobo sauce from chipotle peppers

For the sandwiches:

- 43/4-inch-thick slices sourdough bread
- 1Tbsp butter, softened
- 8oz thinly sliced low-sodium deli ham
- 4ultra-thin slices pepper jack cheese
- Vegetable oil
- 1tsp vinegar
- 4large cold eggs

- Kosher salt
- Ground chipotle powder
- Microgreens or chopped fresh chives

Instructions

1. Preheat oven to 350°F. For the mayo, combine mayonnaise, chipotle chiles, and adobo sauce in a blender or food processor and blend until smooth.
2. For sandwiches, lightly butter both sides of the bread with softened butter. Toast one side of bread in an extra-large oven-proof skillet over medium heat until golden brown. Flip bread slices. While second side is toasting, spread top slice of bread with 1 tablespoon of the mayonnaise. Top with ham and cheese. Transfer pan to oven.
3. While sandwiches are heating, lightly oil the sides of a medium skillet or large saucepan. Fill pan half full with water. Add vinegar to water and bring to a boil.
4. Break 1 egg into a small dish. Carefully slide the egg into the simmering water, holding the lip of the dish as close to the water as possible. Repeat with three remaining eggs, adding them one at a time and spacing them so each egg has an equal amount of

space surrounding it. Simmer for 3 to 5 minutes, or until whites are completely set and yolks begin to thicken but are not hard.

5. Remove sandwiches from oven. Use a slotted spoon to remove eggs from water. Top each sandwich with an egg. Season lightly with salt and chipotle powder. Sprinkle with micro-greens and serve immediately.

6. Note: Refrigerate leftover mayo and use on sandwiches or add it as a topping for steamed or roasted vegetables.

7. Feeling devilish? Ditch the mayo in deviled eggs and swap for creamy avocado in the yolk mixture. This smarter preparation (avocado adds nutrients and healthy monounsaturated fats) makes a powerhouse midday snack or a crowd-pleasing appetizer.

26. Classic Herb Roast Chicken with Root Vegetables

Prep Time: 10 Minutes

Cook Time: 45 Minutes

Servings: 4

Ingredients

- 2 cloves garlic, minced
- 1 Tbsp finely chopped fresh rosemary (Almost any herb works here: thyme, parsley, oregano, basil, or sage)
- Zest and juice of 1 lemon
- 1 Tbsp olive oil
- 1 chicken (4 lb)
- Salt and black pepper to taste
- 1 large russet potato, sliced into 1⁄8" rounds
- 2 onions, quartered
- 4 large carrots, cut into large chunks

Instructions

1. Preheat the oven to 450°F. Mix the garlic, rosemary, lemon zest, and half of the olive oil.
2. Working on the chicken, gently separate the skin from the flesh at the bottom of the breast and spoon in half of the rosemary mixture; use your hands to spread it around as thoroughly as possible.
3. Spread the remaining half over the top of the chicken and then season with plenty of salt and pepper.
4. Mix the potato, onions, carrots, remaining olive oil, and a good pinch of salt and pepper.
5. Arrange the vegetables in the bottom of a roasting pan and place the chicken on top, breast side up.
6. Roast for 20 to 30 minutes, until the skin is lightly browned.
7. Reduce the oven temperature to 350°F and roast for another 30 minutes or so.
8. The chicken is done when the juices between the breast and the leg run clear and an instant-read thermometer inserted deep into the thigh reads 155°F.
9. Remove from the oven and allow to rest for 10 minutes before carving.
10. Serve with the vegetables.

Pre-salting

1. The question of when to salt meat is a subject of much debate in food science circles. Salt draws moisture out, which in theory can dry out a protein. But if you leave it long enough, the moisture will be reabsorbed back into the meat, along with a big shot of seasoning. Rubbing the chicken all over with a teaspoon of kosher salt the night before allows the salt to penetrate all the way to the bone. If you want one way to combat dry, bland chicken, this is it.

27. Beef Stew in Red Wine

Prep Time: 25 Minutes

Cook Time: 55 Minutes

Servings: 8

Ingredients

- 1 Tbsp canola oil
- 3 lb sirloin roast, brisket, or chuck, cut into 1" cubes
- 1 Tbsp flour
- Salt and black pepper to taste
- 2 medium onions, chopped
- 1 cup dry red wine, such as Pinot Noir or Cabernet Sauvignon
- 2 Tbsp tomato paste
- 2 cups chicken broth
- 3 bay leaves
- 8 branches fresh thyme (or 1 tsp dried)
- 6 medium red potatoes, cut into ½" pieces
- 3 medium carrots, peeled and chopped
- 2 cups frozen pearl onions
- 1 cup frozen peas

- Chopped fresh parsley or gremolata

Instructions

2. Heat ½ tablespoon of the oil in a large cast-iron skillet or sauté pan over medium-high heat. Combine the beef and flour in a bowl, season with salt and pepper, and toss to lightly coat the beef.
3. Working in two batches to avoid crowding the pan, sear the beef in the hot oil, turning occasionally, until nicely browned. Transfer to a slow cooker.
4. Add the remaining oil to the skillet.
5. Add the chopped onions and cook for about 5 minutes, until lightly browned.
6. Stir in the wine and tomato paste, scraping the bottom of the pan to free up any browned bits.
7. Pour the onion mixture over the beef, then add the broth, bay leaves, and thyme.
8. Set the slow cooker to high, cover, and cook for about 4 hours (or on low for 8 hours), until the beef is fork-tender.
9. An hour before serving, add the potatoes, carrots, and pearl onions.
10. Five minutes before serving, add the peas.

11. Discard the bay leaves and thyme branches and season with salt and black pepper.

12. Serve garnished with parsley or gremolata if you like.

Eat This Tip

1. While classic beef stew comes with no splashy garnishes, intense meaty dishes like this one are best when finished with a fresh, contrasting note. Cue gremolata, a combination of garlic, parsley, and lemon used to garnish bold Italian dishes like osso buco. The combination also works perfectly on top of grilled steak, roast chicken, and even pasta. To make, combine 2 tablespoons minced garlic with ½ cup minced fresh parsley and 1 tablespoon grated lemon zest.

28. The Best-Ever Healthy Lasagna

Prep Time: 10 Minutes

Cook Time: 55 Minutes

Servings: 8

Ingredients

- 1Tbsp olive oil
- 3links raw chicken sausage, casings removed
- 1small onion, diced
- 2cloves garlic, minced
- Pinch red pepper flakes
- 1can (28 oz) crushed tomatoes
- Salt and black pepper to taste
- 1 1/2 cups low-fat ricotta (Barilla makes a good no-boil lasagna that is widely available.)
- 1/2 cup 2% milk
- 16 sheets no-boil lasagna noodles
- 16–20 fresh basil leaves
- 1cup chopped fresh mozzarella

Instructions

1. Heat the olive oil in a large saucepan over medium heat.
2. Add the sausage and cook for about 3 minutes, until no longer pink.
3. Add the onion, garlic, and red pepper flakes and continue cooking for about 5 minutes, until the onion is soft and translucent.
4. Add the tomatoes and simmer for 15 minutes.
5. Season with salt and pepper.
6. Preheat the oven to 350 degrees Fahrenheit.
7. Combine the ricotta and milk in a mixing bowl.
8. In a 9" x 9" baking pan, lay down a layer of 4 noodles.
9. Cover with a quarter of the ricotta mixture and a quarter of the sausage mixture, then a few basil leaves and a quarter of the mozzarella.
10. Repeat three times to create a four-layer lasagna.
11. Cover with aluminum foil and bake for 25 minutes, until the cheese is melted and the pasta cooked through.
12. Remove the foil and increase the temperature to 450 degrees Fahrenheit.
13. Continue baking for about 10 minutes, until the top of the lasagna is nicely browned.

14. Other ways to layer your lasagna:

15. Sautéed mushrooms and spinach (as many different types as you can find), béchamel, and goat cheese

16. Turkey Bolognese and béchamel with a bit of grated Parmesan on top

29. Healthy Orecchiette with Broccoli Rabe

Prep Time: 15 Minutes

Cook Time: 40 Minutes

Servings: 4

Ingredients

- 1 bunch broccoli rabe, bottom 1" removed
- 10 oz orecchiette pasta
- ½ Tbsp olive oil
- 2 link sun cooked turkey or chicken sausage, casings removed
- 4 cloves garlic, minced
- ¼ tsp red pepper flakes
- ¾ cup low-sodium chicken stock
- Salt and black pepper to taste
- Pecorino Romano or Parmesan

Instructions

1. Bring a large pot of salted water to a boil. Drop in the broccoli rabe and cook for 3 minutes.
2. Use tongs to remove the greens and the chop into ½" pieces.
3. Return the water to a boil. Cook the pasta until al dente.
4. While the pasta cooks, heat the olive oil in a large skillet over medium heat.
5. Add the sausage and cook for about 5 minutes, until lightly browned, then add the garlic and pepper flakes and sauté for another 3 minutes.
6. Stir in the chopped broccoli rabe and chicken stock and lower the heat to a simmer.
7. Season with salt and pepper.
8. Drain the pasta and toss immediately into the pan with the sausage and greens.
9. Toss the pasta (if the mix looks dry, use a bit of the pasta cooking water to loosen it up).
10. Serve immediately with freshly grated cheese.
11. Calorie Cutting:
12. A serving size of pasta in Italy is about 6 ounces; here, many restaurant noodle bowls top 2 pounds. We've used more modest serving sizes for the noodles in the

book's pasta recipes, but kept the sauce portions more substantial. That means the pasta-to-sauce ratio will skew toward the latter, which makes for a more satisfying meal for fewer calories.

30. Rotisserie Chicken Parm Casserole

Prep Time: 20 Minutes

Cook Time: 50 Minutes

Servings: 4

Ingredients

- 8 oz penne or whole wheat pasta, cooked al dente
- 2cups shredded rotisserie chicken
- 11/2 cups tomato sauce
- 1tsp dried parsley
- tsp dried oregano
- 1tsp dried basil
- 1/4 tsp salt
- 1/8 tsp freshly ground black pepper
- 1/8 tsp red pepper flakes
- 1 cup shredded mozzarella cheese (I prefer part-skim)
- 2Tbsp grated Parmesan cheese
- 1/4 cup Italian-style bread crumbs

Instructions

1. Preheat the oven to 350°F. Coat an 8-inch square baking dish with nonstick cooking spray.

2. In a medium bowl, toss together the pasta, chicken, 1 cup of the tomato sauce, parsley, oregano, basil, salt, black pepper, and red pepper flakes.

3. Spoon the mixture into the prepared baking dish. Top the casserole with the remaining 1/2 cup tomato sauce and spread evenly with the back of a spoon. Sprinkle evenly with the mozzarella cheese, Parmesan cheese, and bread crumbs.

4. Bake until the top is bubbly and golden brown, about 25 minutes.